# The Ultimate Guide to **Pregnancy**:

## A Comprehensive Resource for Women

Gracjan Krzeszowiec

# 1. INTRODUCTION TO PREGNANCY

Pregnancy is a miraculous and transformative time in a woman's life. It is a time of growth, change, and anticipation, as a woman's body nourishes and supports the development of a new life. However, pregnancy can also bring many challenges, both physical and emotional. In this chapter, we will discuss the stages of pregnancy, common pregnancy symptoms and discomforts, and an overview of prenatal care.

**Understanding the stages of pregnancy:**

Pregnancy is typically divided into three trimesters, each lasting approximately 12-14 weeks. The first trimester begins on the first day of a woman's last menstrual period and lasts until the end of the 13th week of pregnancy. The second trimester lasts from week 14 to week 27, while the third trimester spans from week 28 until the end of pregnancy.

During each trimester, a woman's body undergoes significant changes to support the growth and development of the fetus.

These changes include hormonal fluctuations, increased blood volume, and physical changes to the uterus, cervix, and other reproductive organs.

**Pregnancy can also bring a variety of uncomfortable symptoms and discomforts, including:**

- **Morning sickness:** nausea and vomiting, especially in the first trimester.

- **Fatigue:** feeling tired or exhausted, often due to hormonal changes.

- **Constipation:** difficulty passing bowel movements due to slowed digestion.

- **Heartburn:** burning sensation in the chest due to increased stomach acid.

- **Back pain:** pain in the lower back due to increased weight and changes in posture.
- Swelling: swelling in the feet and ankles due to fluid retention.

- **Braxton hicks contractions:** painless contractions that prepare the uterus for labor.

It is important for women to communicate any discomforts or symptoms they are experiencing with their healthcare provider, who can offer advice and recommendations for relief.

Prenatal care is a critical component of a healthy pregnancy. It involves regular check-ups with a healthcare provider to monitor the health and development of the fetus, as well as the mother's health. Prenatal care typically includes:

- **Physical exams:** the healthcare provider will perform routine physical exams, including blood pressure and weight checks, to monitor the mother's health.

- **Ultrasound exams:** ultrasound exams are used to monitor fetal growth and development, as well as detect any potential complications.

- **Prenatal testing:** prenatal testing may be recommended based on the mother's age, medical history, or other factors. This may include genetic testing, screening for gestational diabetes, or other tests to monitor fetal health.

- **Nutritional counseling:** a healthcare provider can offer advice on healthy eating habits during pregnancy, including recommendations for supplements such as folic acid and iron.

- **Education and support:** prenatal care may also involve education and support on topics such as childbirth preparation, breastfeeding, and postpartum recovery.

It is important for women to prioritize prenatal care throughout their pregnancy to ensure the health and well-being of themselves and their baby.

# 2. PREPARING FOR PREGNANCY

Preparing for pregnancy is an important step in ensuring a healthy pregnancy and a healthy baby. In this chapter, we will discuss important steps to take before getting pregnant, including lifestyle changes, prenatal testing, and fertility considerations.

Before getting pregnant, it is important to make healthy lifestyle changes to prepare your body for pregnancy. Some important changes to consider include:

- **Eating a healthy diet:** A well-balanced diet that includes fruits, vegetables, whole grains, lean proteins, and healthy fats is important for the health of both you and your baby.

- **Getting regular exercise:** Regular exercise can help prepare your body for the physical demands of pregnancy and childbirth. It is important to consult with your healthcare provider about the type and amount of exercise that is safe during pregnancy.

- **Quitting smoking and avoiding alcohol and drugs:** Smoking, alcohol, and drugs can harm both you and your developing baby. It is important to quit smoking and avoid alcohol and drugs before getting pregnant.

- **Managing chronic conditions:** If you have a chronic condition such as diabetes, hypertension, or thyroid disease, it is important to work with your healthcare provider to manage the condition before getting pregnant.

It is also important to consider prenatal testing. Prenatal testing can help identify potential health concerns for you or your baby, allowing for early intervention and treatment.

- **Genetic testing:** Genetic testing can help identify the risk of certain genetic disorders. This may involve testing for inherited conditions such as cystic fibrosis or sickle cell disease, or screening for chromosomal abnormalities such as Down syndrome.

- **Infectious disease testing:** Testing for infectious diseases such as HIV, hepatitis B and C, and sexually transmitted infections (STIs) can help identify potential risks for the mother and baby.

- **Medical history review:** A review of your medical history can help identify potential risks for you and your baby, such as previous miscarriages, stillbirths, or preterm labor.

If you are having difficulty getting pregnant, it may be helpful to consider fertility treatments or interventions.

**Some options to consider include:**

- **Fertility medications:** Medications that stimulate ovulation can increase the chances of pregnancy for women who are having difficulty conceiving.

- **Assisted reproductive technology (ART):** ART includes procedures such as in vitro fertilization (IVF), which can help increase the chances of pregnancy for couples who are experiencing infertility.

- **Surgery:** In some cases, surgical interventions may be necessary to address fertility issues, such as removing fibroids or repairing damaged fallopian tubes.

Preparing for pregnancy involves making important lifestyle changes, considering prenatal testing, and addressing any fertility concerns.

**By taking these steps, you can increase the likelihood of a healthy pregnancy and a healthy baby.**

# 3. FIRST TRIMESTER (WEEKS 1–12)

The first trimester of pregnancy is a time of significant physical and emotional changes for both the mother and the developing fetus. In this chapter, we will discuss the major milestones and changes that occur during the first trimester, as well as important steps to take for a healthy pregnancy.

**Weeks 1–4: Conception and Implantation**

During the first week of pregnancy, fertilization occurs when the sperm meets the egg in the fallopian tube. The fertilized egg then travels down the fallopian tube towards the uterus, dividing rapidly into multiple cells. By the end of the first week, the fertilized egg has developed into a ball of cells called a blastocyst.

During the second week, the blastocyst reaches the uterus and implants into the uterine lining. The blastocyst then begins to form two distinct layers: the inner cell mass, which will develop into the embryo, and the outer layer, which will develop into the placenta.

**Weeks 5-8: development of the embryo**

During the third week of pregnancy, the inner cell mass begins to develop into the embryo. The embryo begins to form a neural tube, which will eventually develop into the brain and spinal cord. The heart also begins to form and starts to beat by the end of the fourth week.

During the fifth week, the embryo begins to develop major organs and structures, including the liver, lungs, and digestive system. The head and facial features also begin to take shape.

By the end of the eighth week, the embryo is about an inch long and has developed most of its major organs and structures. The embryo is now called a fetus.

**Weeks 9-12: maturation of the fetus**

During the ninth week, the fetus's major organs and structures continue to mature and develop. The fingers and toes become fully formed, and the fetal heartbeat can now be heard using a doppler device.

During the tenth and eleventh weeks, the fetus begins to develop reflexes, including the ability to suck and swallow. The fetus also begins to move around more and can be seen on an ultrasound.

By the end of the twelfth week, the fetus is about two and a half inches long and weighs about half an ounce. The fetus's sex organs have also developed, although it may be too early to determine the sex on an ultrasound.

# 4. SECOND TRIMESTER (WEEKS 13-27)

The second trimester is often considered the "honeymoon phase" of pregnancy, as many women experience relief from the early symptoms of pregnancy and begin to feel more energetic and comfortable. In this chapter, we will discuss the major milestones and changes that occur during the second trimester, as well as important steps to take for a healthy pregnancy.

**Weeks 13-16: Growth and Movement**

During the thirteenth week of pregnancy, the fetus is about three inches long and weighs about an ounce. The fetus's arms and legs continue to grow, and the fingers and toes now have nails. The fetus's vocal cords also begin to develop.

During the fourteenth and fifteenth weeks, the fetus begins to move around more, and the mother may start to feel "fluttering" sensations in her belly.
By the end of the sixteenth week, the fetus is about four and a half inches long and weighs about three ounces. The fetus's skin is still thin and translucent, and the sex can often be determined on an ultrasound.

**Weeks 17-20: Sensory Development**

During the seventeenth week of pregnancy, the fetus's hearing and vision begin to develop. The fetus can now hear sounds outside the womb, including the mother's voice and other noises.

During the eighteenth and nineteenth weeks, the fetus's sense of touch and taste begin to develop. The fetus may start to suck its thumb and can now distinguish between sweet and bitter tastes.

By the end of the twentieth week, the fetus is about six and a half inches long and weighs about ten ounces. The mother may now feel the fetus's movements more distinctly and regularly.

**Weeks 21–24: Lung Development**

During the twenty-first week of pregnancy, the fetus's lungs begin to produce surfactant, a substance that helps the lungs expand and contract. The fetus's digestive system also begins to produce meconium, the first bowel movement.
During the twenty-second and twenty-third weeks, the fetus's brain continues to develop rapidly, and the fetus's sense of touch becomes even more sensitive.

By the end of the twenty-fourth week, the fetus is about a foot long and weighs about a pound and a half. The fetus's skin is less translucent, and the fetus can now blink and make facial expressions.

**Weeks 25–27: Viability**

During the twenty-fifth week of pregnancy, the fetus's eyes begin to open and close, and the fetus's blood vessels in the lungs begin to expand. The fetus also begins to develop fat deposits, which will help regulate body temperature after birth.

During the twenty-sixth and twenty-seventh weeks, the fetus's lungs continue to develop, and the fetus's brain continues to mature.

By the end of the twenty-seventh week, the fetus is about fourteen inches long and weighs about two pounds. At this point, the fetus is considered "viable," meaning it has a chance of survival outside the womb with medical intervention.

# 5. THIRD TRIMESTER (WEEKS 28-40)

The third trimester is the final stretch of pregnancy and is a time of significant growth and development for both the fetus and the mother. In this chapter, we will discuss the major milestones and changes that occur during the third trimester, as well as important steps to take for a healthy pregnancy and preparation for childbirth.

**Weeks 28-32: Fetal Growth and Development**

During the twenty-eighth week of pregnancy, the fetus is about fourteen and a half inches long and weighs about two and a half pounds. The fetus's eyes can now track light and the fetus can distinguish between light and dark.

During the twenty-ninth and thirtieth weeks, the fetus's bones continue to harden, and the fetus's brain continues to develop rapidly. The fetus's hearing is also well-developed, and it can now recognize the mother's voice.

By the end of the thirty-second week, the fetus is about sixteen and a half inches long and weighs about four pounds. The fetus's body is becoming more proportionate, and the fetus is now capable of regulating its own body temperature.

## Weeks 33–36: Fetal Positioning and Preparation for Birth

During the thirty-third week of pregnancy, the fetus is about seventeen and a half inches long and weighs about five pounds. The fetus's head is usually facing down towards the cervix in preparation for birth.

During the thirty-fourth and thirty-fifth weeks, the fetus continues to gain weight and may start to experience less space in the womb. The mother may feel more pressure on her pelvic area and experience Braxton Hicks contractions.

By the end of the thirty-sixth week, the fetus is about eighteen and a half inches long and weighs about six pounds. The fetus's lungs are nearly fully developed, and the fetus is now considered "early-term" and has a good chance of survival if born prematurely.

## Weeks 37–40: Full-Term and Preparation for Birth

During the thirty-seventh and thirty-eighth weeks of pregnancy, the fetus's major organs are fully developed, and the fetus continues to gain weight and size. The mother may start to experience more frequent and stronger contractions.

By the end of the thirty-ninth week, the fetus is considered "full-term," meaning it is ready for birth. The fetus is about twenty inches long and weighs about seven and a half pounds. The mother may experience signs of labor, such as the breaking of her water or regular contractions.

**During these three trimesters, there are several important steps to take to ensure a healthy pregnancy and preparation for childbirth, including:**

- **Prenatal care:** Continuing to receive regular prenatal care is important for monitoring the fetus's growth and development and identifying any potential risks or concerns.

- **Healthy lifestyle choices:** Continuing to eat a healthy diet, getting regular exercise, and avoiding alcohol, tobacco, and drugs are important for a healthy pregnancy and preparation for birth.

- **Birth plan:** Creating a birth plan with the healthcare provider can help ensure a positive birth experience and communicate preferences for pain management and other aspects of childbirth.

- **Preparing for labor:** Taking childbirth education classes and practicing relaxation and breathing techniques can help prepare the mother for labor and delivery.

- **Mental health:** Taking care of mental health and seeking support from loved ones or healthcare providers can help manage the stress and emotional challenges of pregnancy and childbirth.

- **Postpartum planning:** Planning for postpartum care, including childcare, recovery, and support, can help ease the transition into parenthood.

# 6. NUTRITION AND EXERCISE DURING PREGNANCY

Pregnancy is a time when a woman's body undergoes significant changes, and it's important to prioritize good nutrition and exercise to support a healthy pregnancy and baby. In this chapter, we'll explore the key components of a healthy pregnancy diet and the benefits of regular exercise during pregnancy.

**Nutrition During Pregnancy:**

A healthy pregnancy diet should include a variety of nutrient-rich foods to support the growth and development of the fetus. Some key nutrients to focus on include:

- **Protein:** Protein is essential for fetal growth and development and should make up around 25% of a pregnant woman's daily caloric intake. Good sources of protein include lean meats, poultry, fish, beans, lentils, and dairy products.

- **Folate:** Folate is critical for the development of the fetus's nervous system and can help prevent neural tube defects. Good sources of folate include leafy greens, fortified cereals, beans, and citrus fruits.

- **Iron:** Iron is necessary for the production of red blood cells and is essential for fetal growth and development. Good sources of iron include lean meats, poultry, fish, beans, lentils, and fortified cereals.

- **Calcium:** Calcium is important for the development of the fetus's bones and teeth. Good sources of calcium include dairy products, leafy greens, and fortified cereals.

- **Omega-3 fatty acids:** Omega-3 fatty acids are important for fetal brain and eye development. Good sources of omega-3 fatty acids include fatty fish, nuts, and seeds.

It's also important to stay hydrated during pregnancy, aiming for at least eight glasses of water per day. Pregnant women should avoid certain foods, including raw or undercooked meat, fish with high levels of mercury, raw or undercooked eggs, and unpasteurized dairy products.

**Exercise During Pregnancy:**

Regular exercise during pregnancy can help support a healthy pregnancy, reduce the risk of complications, and promote a faster recovery after childbirth.
Some of the benefits of exercise during pregnancy include:

- **Improved cardiovascular health:** Regular exercise can help improve cardiovascular health and reduce the risk of gestational diabetes and preeclampsia.

- **Improved mood:** Exercise can help boost mood and reduce stress and anxiety.

- **Improved sleep:** Regular exercise can help improve sleep quality during pregnancy.

- **Easier labor and delivery:** Exercise during pregnancy can help improve endurance and strength, making labor and delivery easier.

- **Faster postpartum recovery:** Women who exercise during pregnancy often experience a faster postpartum recovery.

Some good forms of exercise during pregnancy include walking, swimming, yoga, and low-impact aerobics. Pregnant women should avoid high-impact activities, contact sports, and activities with a high risk of falling.

It's important to consult with a healthcare provider before starting or continuing an exercise program during pregnancy, especially if there are any underlying health concerns or complications.

In conclusion, good nutrition and exercise are essential for a healthy pregnancy and baby. Pregnant women should focus on eating a nutrient-rich diet and staying hydrated, while also incorporating regular exercise into their routine.

**Consulting with a healthcare provider can help ensure a safe and effective nutrition and exercise plan during pregnancy.**

# 7.MANAGING PREGNANCY COMPLICATIONS

While pregnancy is generally a healthy and natural process, some women may experience complications that require medical attention. In this chapter, we'll explore some of the most common pregnancy complications and how they can be managed.

- **Gestational diabetes:** Gestational diabetes is a type of diabetes that occurs during pregnancy. It can cause high blood sugar levels, which can lead to complications for both the mother and baby. Treatment may involve monitoring blood sugar levels, modifying the diet, and, in some cases, taking medication.

- **Preeclampsia:** Preeclampsia is a serious condition that can occur in the second half of pregnancy. It's characterized by high blood pressure and damage to organs such as the liver and kidneys. Treatment may involve medication to lower blood pressure, bed rest, and early delivery if necessary.

- **Preterm labor:** Preterm labor is when contractions begin before 37 weeks of pregnancy. It can be caused by a variety of factors, including infection, stress, and certain medical conditions. Treatment may involve bed rest, medication to stop contractions, or an early delivery.

- **Miscarriage:** Miscarriage is the loss of a pregnancy before 20 weeks. It can be caused by a variety of factors, including chromosomal abnormalities, infections, and medical conditions. Treatment may involve monitoring, medication to help pass the tissue, or a surgical procedure.

- **Ectopic pregnancy:** Ectopic pregnancy occurs when the fertilized egg implants outside the uterus, typically in the fallopian tube. It can be life-threatening if left untreated. Treatment may involve medication to dissolve the pregnancy, laparoscopic surgery to remove the pregnancy, or emergency surgery in severe cases.

- **Placenta previa:** Placenta previa is when the placenta covers the cervix, making vaginal delivery impossible. Treatment may involve bed rest, medication to control bleeding, or a cesarean delivery.
- **Group B streptococcus:** Group B streptococcus is a type of bacterial infection that can be passed from the mother to the baby during delivery. Treatment may involve antibiotics during labor and delivery to prevent transmission to the baby.

**If a woman experiences any of these complications during pregnancy, it's important to seek medical attention promptly.**

Treatment options may vary depending on the severity of the complication and the health of the mother and baby.

In some cases, close monitoring and management may be enough, while in other cases, more aggressive treatment may be necessary.

In conclusion, while most pregnancies are healthy and uncomplicated, some women may experience complications that require medical attention. By understanding the signs and symptoms of common pregnancy complications and seeking medical attention promptly, women can take steps to manage these complications and support a healthy pregnancy and baby.

# 8. EMOTIONAL AND MENTAL HEALTH DURING PREGNANCY

Pregnancy can be an exciting and joyful time, but it can also be a time of stress and anxiety. In this chapter, we'll explore the emotional and mental health aspects of pregnancy and provide tips for managing stress and maintaining a healthy mindset.

- **Mood changes:** It's common for women to experience mood changes during pregnancy, including anxiety, depression, and irritability. These changes are often related to hormonal fluctuations, but other factors, such as stress and lifestyle changes, can also play a role.

- **Coping with stress:** Pregnancy can be a stressful time, with physical, emotional, and social changes happening all at once. It's important to find healthy ways to cope with stress, such as exercise, meditation, deep breathing, or talking with friends or a therapist.

- **Building a support system:** A strong support system can be essential for managing the emotional ups and downs of pregnancy. This may include family, friends, a partner, or a support group.

- **Self-care:** Taking care of oneself during pregnancy is essential for both physical and emotional health. This may include getting enough rest, eating a healthy diet, practicing good hygiene, and finding time for relaxation and enjoyable activities.

- **Mental health conditions:** Women who have a history of mental health conditions, such as depression or anxiety, may be at increased risk of experiencing these conditions during pregnancy. It's important to discuss any concerns with a healthcare provider and develop a plan for managing mental health during pregnancy.

- **Postpartum depression:** Postpartum depression is a type of depression that occurs after giving birth. It's important for women to be aware of the symptoms and risk factors for postpartum depression and to seek help if needed.

- **Seeking professional help:** If a woman is experiencing significant stress, anxiety, or depression during pregnancy, it's important to seek professional help. This may include talking with a therapist, psychiatrist, or other mental health professional.

In conclusion, pregnancy can be a time of emotional and mental ups and downs, and it's important for women to prioritize their mental health during this time.

By building a strong support system, practicing self-care, and seeking professional help if needed, women can manage stress and maintain a healthy mindset throughout pregnancy and beyond.

# 9. LABOR AND DELIVERY

Labor and delivery are the culmination of the pregnancy journey, and it's important for women to be informed and prepared for this life-changing event. In this chapter, we'll explore the stages of labor and delivery, common interventions, and postpartum recovery.

- **Signs of labor:** labor can begin with a range of symptoms, including contractions, vaginal bleeding, and rupture of the amniotic sac. Women should be aware of the signs of labor and contact their healthcare provider if they have any concerns.

- **Stages of labor:** labor is typically divided into three stages: the early stage, active stage, and pushing stage. During these stages, the cervix will gradually dilate, and the baby will move through the birth canal.

- **Pain management:** labor can be painful, and women have a range of options for managing pain during labor, including breathing techniques, relaxation, hydrotherapy, massage, and medication.

- **Medical interventions:** in some cases, medical interventions may be necessary during labor, including induction of labor, assisted delivery (such as forceps or vacuum extraction), or cesarean delivery (c-section). Women should discuss their preferences for medical interventions with their healthcare provider.

- **Delivery:** once the baby is born, the healthcare provider will clamp and cut the umbilical cord, and the placenta will be delivered. The healthcare provider will then perform a newborn assessment and check the mother for any tears or other injuries.

- **Postpartum recovery:** after delivery, women will need time to recover and adjust to their new role as a mother. This may include physical recovery from delivery, breastfeeding challenges, and emotional adjustments.

- **Postpartum care:** women should receive regular postpartum care from their healthcare provider to monitor for any complications and provide support for breastfeeding, mental health, and other postpartum concerns.

In conclusion, labor and delivery can be a daunting experience, but with preparation, support, and informed decision-making, women can have a positive birth experience.

By understanding the stages of labor, pain management options, medical interventions, and postpartum recovery, women can feel empowered and confident in their ability to give birth.

# 10.POSTPARTUM RECOVERY

After giving birth, women undergo significant physical and emotional changes as they recover and adjust to their new role as a mother. In this chapter, we'll explore the physical and emotional aspects of postpartum recovery and provide tips for managing this important time.

- **Physical recovery:** After giving birth, women will experience physical changes such as vaginal bleeding, soreness, and breast engorgement. It's important to get enough rest, eat a healthy diet, and stay hydrated to support physical recovery.

- **Breastfeeding:** Breastfeeding can be a rewarding experience, but it can also be challenging. Women should seek support from a lactation consultant or other breastfeeding expert to ensure successful breastfeeding.

- **Postpartum exercise:** Exercise can help women regain their strength and energy after giving birth. Women should discuss with their healthcare provider about when it's safe to start exercising and what types of activities are appropriate.

- **Emotional recovery**: The postpartum period can be emotionally challenging, with feelings of joy, exhaustion, anxiety, and depression. It's important to talk about these emotions with a partner, family member, friend, or healthcare provider.

- **Bonding with the baby:** Bonding with the baby is an essential aspect of the postpartum period. Women should spend time holding, cuddling, and interacting with their baby to foster a strong bond.

- **Sleep deprivation:** Sleep deprivation is a common experience for new mothers. Women should prioritize sleep when possible and ask for help from a partner, family member, or friend to get rest when needed.

- **Postpartum depression:** Postpartum depression is a type of depression that occurs after giving birth. It's important to be aware of the symptoms and seek help if necessary.

- **Sexual health:** Women should wait until they have been cleared by their healthcare provider before resuming sexual activity. It's important to communicate with a partner about any concerns and take time to adjust to changes in sexual function and desire.

In conclusion, postpartum recovery is a crucial period for women as they recover from the physical and emotional changes of giving birth.

By taking care of their physical health, seeking emotional support, bonding with the baby, and communicating with a partner about sexual health, women can navigate this important time with confidence and grace.

# 11. POSTPARTUM DEPRESSION

The postpartum period is a time of significant adjustment for new mothers. While many women experience joy and excitement after giving birth, others may experience feelings of sadness, anxiety, or overwhelm. Postpartum depression and anxiety are common conditions that affect many new mothers during this time. In this chapter, we will explore postpartum depression and anxiety in detail, including their symptoms, causes, and treatments.

**Understanding Postpartum Depression and Anxiety:**

Postpartum depression (PPD) is a mood disorder that can affect women after childbirth. Symptoms of PPD include feelings of sadness, hopelessness, and worthlessness. Women with PPD may also experience changes in appetite, sleep disturbances, and difficulty bonding with their baby. Postpartum anxiety is another condition that can affect new mothers. Symptoms of postpartum anxiety (PPA) can include constant worry, restlessness, and physical symptoms such as sweating or heart palpitations.

Women who experience symptoms of PPD or PPA should talk to their healthcare provider or a mental health professional for support and treatment.

Postpartum depression and anxiety are common conditions that affect many women during the postpartum period.

Recognizing the signs and symptoms of these conditions, as well as understanding the risk factors and treatment options, can be an important part of promoting mental health and well-being for new mothers.

By seeking help and support, women can better manage their symptoms and enjoy a positive postpartum experience.

# 12. NEWBORN CARE

After months of preparation and anticipation, your little one has finally arrived! Taking care of a newborn can be both exciting and overwhelming, especially if it's your first time. In this chapter, we'll provide a comprehensive guide to newborn care to help you navigate this important time.

- **Feeding:** Whether you choose to breastfeed or formula-feed, feeding your baby is a top priority. Newborns need to eat every 2-3 hours, so it's important to establish a feeding routine and watch for signs of hunger.

- **Sleep:** Newborns sleep a lot, but they also wake up frequently to eat. It's important to establish a safe sleeping environment, such as placing your baby on their back in a crib with no soft objects or loose bedding.

- **Diapering:** Newborns need frequent diaper changes, typically every 2-3 hours. Be sure to have plenty of diapers, wipes, and diaper rash cream on hand.

- **Bathing:** Newborns don't need to be bathed every day, but it's important to keep their face, neck, hands, and diaper area clean. Use a gentle, unscented soap and warm water.

- **Soothing:** Newborns cry to communicate their needs, but it can be difficult to determine what they want. Try different soothing techniques, such as swaddling, rocking, or singing, to see what works best for your baby.

- **Developmental milestones:** Although newborns can't do much, they will begin to reach developmental milestones such as lifting their head, making eye contact, and smiling. Track your baby's milestones and discuss any concerns with your healthcare provider.

- **Safety:** Newborns are fragile and need to be protected from hazards such as choking, suffocation, and falls. Be sure to follow safety guidelines, such as using a car seat and keeping hazardous objects out of reach.

- **Healthcare:** Newborns need to see a pediatrician regularly for check-ups and vaccinations. Be sure to schedule appointments and ask any questions you have about your baby's health.

In conclusion, taking care of a newborn can be a challenging but rewarding experience. By prioritizing feeding and sleeping, keeping your baby clean and safe, tracking developmental milestones, and seeking healthcare when necessary, you can provide the best care for your little one.

**Remember to take care of yourself too, as being a new parent can be exhausting both physically and emotionally.**

# 13.BREASTFEEDING

Breastfeeding is a natural and healthy way to nourish a newborn baby. It provides many benefits for both the mother and the baby, including essential nutrients and antibodies that help protect against infections and diseases. This chapter will provide a comprehensive guide to breastfeeding, covering the benefits of breastfeeding, different techniques and positions, common challenges, pumping and storing breast milk, and introducing solid foods.

**Benefits of Breastfeeding:**

Breastfeeding provides many benefits for both the mother and the baby. For the baby, breast milk contains all the essential nutrients and antibodies needed for healthy growth and development. It also helps protect against infections, such as ear infections, respiratory infections, and gastrointestinal infections. Breastfeeding has also been shown to reduce the risk of sudden infant death syndrome (SIDS) and certain childhood cancers.

For the mother, breastfeeding helps the uterus return to its pre-pregnancy size, reduces the risk of postpartum bleeding, and may lower the risk of breast and ovarian cancer.

Breastfeeding also promotes bonding between the mother and the baby, and can provide a sense of emotional satisfaction and fulfillment.

**Techniques and Positions:**

There are several different techniques and positions for breastfeeding, and it is important for new mothers to find the one that works best for them and their baby. Some popular positions include:

- **Cradle hold:** This is a classic position where the baby lies across the mother's lap with the baby's head resting in the crook of the mother's arm.

- **Football hold:** This position is where the baby is held under the arm like a football, with the mother's hand supporting the baby's head and neck.

- **Side-lying position:** This position is where the mother and baby lie on their sides facing each other, with the baby's head at the level of the mother's breast.

**Common Challenges:**

While breastfeeding is a natural process, it can come with some challenges for new mothers. Some common challenges include sore nipples, engorgement, and low milk supply.

Sore nipples can occur when the baby is not latching properly or when the baby is not feeding often enough. Applying a lanolin cream or other nipple cream can help alleviate the pain.

Engorgement occurs when the breasts become overly full and can be painful. Massaging the breasts before and during feeding, and applying a warm compress to the breasts can help relieve engorgement.

Low milk supply can occur due to stress, dehydration, or not breastfeeding often enough. Taking steps to reduce stress, staying hydrated, and feeding the baby on demand can help increase milk supply.

**Pumping and Storing Breast Milk:**

Sometimes, new mothers may need to pump and store breast milk for times when they are away from their baby. This can be done using a manual or electric breast pump.

The stored milk can be kept in a refrigerator or freezer for later use. It is important to follow proper storage guidelines and to use the oldest milk first.

**Introducing Solid Foods:**

When the baby is ready, usually around 6 months of age, solid foods can be introduced in addition to breastfeeding. It is important to introduce solid foods gradually and to choose age-appropriate foods. Some good first foods include mashed fruits and vegetables, rice cereal, and pureed meats.

Breastfeeding is a natural and healthy way to nourish a newborn baby. It provides many benefits for both the mother and the baby, and can promote bonding between them. While it may come with some challenges, with the right techniques and support, most new mothers can successfully breastfeed their babies.

# 14. FORMULA FEEDING

While breastfeeding is considered the gold standard for infant nutrition, formula feeding is a common choice for many families. Formula feeding can provide all the necessary nutrients that babies need to grow and thrive, and can be a viable option for mothers who are unable or choose not to breastfeed.

**Types of Formula:**

There are many different types of formula available, including cow's milk-based formula, soy-based formula, and hypoallergenic formula. Each type of formula has different advantages and disadvantages, and it is important to discuss with a pediatrician which type of formula is best for your baby.

**How to Prepare Formula:**

Proper preparation of formula is crucial to ensure that babies receive the right amount of nutrients and that the formula is free from harmful bacteria. Formula should always be prepared according to the instructions on the package, using the correct amount of water and powder.

**Feeding Schedule:**

Newborns typically feed every 2-3 hours, and the amount of formula they need will vary depending on their age and weight. It is important to pay attention to baby's hunger cues and feed on demand, rather than on a strict schedule.

**Bottle-feeding Techniques:**

Proper bottle-feeding techniques can help prevent gas, colic, and other digestive issues in babies. These techniques include holding the baby in an upright position, allowing for frequent burping, and ensuring that the baby's mouth is properly sealed around the nipple.

**Sterilization and Cleaning:**

Bottles, nipples, and other feeding accessories should be thoroughly cleaned and sterilized before each use to prevent the spread of bacteria. This can be done by boiling items in water or using a sterilizer.

## Switching to Solid Foods:

 Most babies begin eating solid foods around 6 months of age, although this can vary. It is important to introduce new foods gradually and to continue offering formula or breast milk until the baby is ready to transition fully to solid foods.

## Working and Formula Feeding:

Many working mothers choose to formula feed their babies due to the convenience of having the baby's caregiver provide the formula during the day. It is important to communicate with caregivers about proper feeding techniques and to have a plan for storing and transporting formula.

While breastfeeding is the recommended method of infant feeding, formula feeding can also be a safe and healthy option for babies.

With proper preparation and feeding techniques, formula feeding can provide all the necessary nutrients that babies need to grow and thrive. It is important to discuss any concerns or questions with a pediatrician to ensure that your baby is getting the best possible nutrition.

# 15. RETURNING TO WORK AND PARENTING

Returning to work after having a baby can be a difficult and emotional transition for many parents. Balancing the demands of work and parenting can be challenging, but with planning and preparation, it is possible to navigate this time successfully. In this chapter, we will provide a detailed guide to help new parents prepare for their return to work and manage the ongoing demands of parenting.

- **Planning for childcare:** Finding the right childcare provider is crucial to a smooth transition back to work. Options include daycare centers, family daycare, in-home providers, or nannies. Research your options carefully and choose a provider that aligns with your values and needs.

- **Managing schedules:** Juggling work and parenting schedules can be challenging.

Be sure to communicate with your employer and childcare provider to establish a consistent routine that works for everyone.

- **Maintaining a healthy work-life balance:** It's important to prioritize self-care and maintain a healthy work-life balance. Set realistic expectations for yourself and learn to delegate responsibilities where possible.

- **Breastfeeding and pumping:** If you plan to breastfeed, it's important to have a plan in place for pumping at work. Speak with your employer about your rights to breaks and a private space to pump.

- **Staying connected with your child:** It's important to stay connected with your child even while you are at work. Consider setting up regular video calls or leaving notes for your child's caregiver.

- **Seeking support:** It can be helpful to connect with other parents who are also balancing work and parenting.

Seek out support groups or online forums to share experiences and gain tips and advice.

- **Managing guilt:** It's common for parents to experience guilt when returning to work. Remember that taking care of your own needs and providing for your family is an important part of parenting.

- **Managing finances:** Balancing the costs of childcare and the demands of work can be financially challenging. Consider creating a budget and exploring options for flexible work schedules or additional income streams.

In conclusion, returning to work after having a baby is a major life transition. By planning for childcare, managing schedules, prioritizing self-care, maintaining a connection with your child, seeking support, managing guilt, and managing finances, you can successfully balance the demands of work and parenting. Remember to be patient with yourself and seek help when needed.

# 16. SPECIAL CONSIDERATIONS FOR PREGNANCY

While pregnancy is a natural process, there are some special considerations that may arise for some women. In this chapter, we will explore some of the most common special considerations for pregnancy, including high-risk pregnancies, multiple gestations, and advanced maternal age.

- High-risk pregnancies: A high-risk pregnancy is one in which the health of the mother or baby is at risk due to pre-existing conditions or complications that arise during pregnancy. These may include conditions such as diabetes, high blood pressure, or gestational diabetes. Women with high-risk pregnancies may require closer monitoring and medical intervention to ensure the health of both mother and baby.

- Multiple gestations: Women carrying more than one fetus, such as twins or triplets, may require additional monitoring and care. These pregnancies may be more likely to result in preterm labor, gestational diabetes, or preeclampsia. Close monitoring and early intervention can help ensure the health of both mother and babies.

- Advanced maternal age: Women who become pregnant at age 35 or older are considered to have an advanced maternal age pregnancy. These pregnancies may be more likely to result in complications such as gestational diabetes, high blood pressure, or preterm labor. Women with advanced maternal age pregnancies may require closer monitoring and medical intervention to ensure the health of both mother and baby.

- Preterm labor: Preterm labor is labor that occurs before the 37th week of pregnancy. This can be a serious concern as premature babies may require additional medical care and have a higher risk of long-term health problems. Women who experience preterm labor may require medical intervention to help prevent early delivery.

- Infections: Some infections can be particularly harmful to pregnant women and their developing fetuses. These may include infections such as cytomegalovirus (CMV), listeria, or Zika virus. Women should take precautions to avoid exposure to these infections and seek medical care if they suspect they have been exposed.

- Pre-eclampsia: Pre-eclampsia is a serious condition that can occur during pregnancy, characterized by high blood pressure and damage to organs such as the liver or kidneys. It can be life-threatening if left untreated. Women who develop pre-eclampsia may require close monitoring and medical intervention to ensure the health of both mother and baby.

In conclusion, while pregnancy is a natural process, there are some special considerations that may arise for some women. High-risk pregnancies, multiple gestations, advanced maternal age, preterm labor, infections, and pre-eclampsia are all concerns that may require additional monitoring and medical intervention.

It's important for women to be aware of these risks and to seek medical care if they suspect they may be experiencing complications. Close monitoring and early intervention can help ensure the health of both mother and baby.

# 17. PREGNANCY AND SEXUALITY

Pregnancy is a time of great physical and emotional changes, and many expectant parents may wonder about how their sexuality will be affected during this time. In this chapter, we will explore the ways that pregnancy can impact sexual health and relationships, and offer tips for navigating these changes.

During pregnancy, a woman's body undergoes significant physical changes that can affect sexual health and comfort. Some common physical changes during pregnancy include:

- Increased blood flow to the pelvic area, which can result in more sensitive and engorged genitalia.

- Changes in hormone levels, which can cause changes in libido and sexual desire.

- Nausea, fatigue, and other symptoms of pregnancy that can decrease sexual desire and energy.

- Physical discomfort or pain during sex due to changes in the cervix or uterus, or pressure on the bladder or other organs.

**Navigating sexual changes during pregnancy:**

Many couples experience changes in their sexual relationship during pregnancy, and it's important to communicate openly and honestly with each other about these changes. Here are some tips for navigating sexual changes during pregnancy:

Talk openly with your partner about how you're feeling and what you need. Don't be afraid to ask for what you want, or to say no if you're not comfortable.

Explore different sexual positions or activities that are comfortable and safe during pregnancy. Many couples find that side-lying positions or manual stimulation can be more comfortable than traditional penetrative sex.

Experiment with non-sexual intimacy, such as cuddling, massage, or other forms of touch. These activities can help maintain intimacy and connection during times when sexual activity may be less desirable or comfortable.

Be patient with yourself and your partner, and recognize that changes in sexual desire or comfort are normal and may vary throughout the pregnancy.

**Sexual health and safety during pregnancy:**

It's important to take steps to maintain sexual health and safety during pregnancy. Some things to keep in mind include:

Communicate openly with your healthcare provider about any sexual concerns or questions you may have.

Use protection, such as condoms or dental dams, to prevent the transmission of sexually transmitted infections (STIs) during pregnancy.

Avoid activities that could increase the risk of injury or trauma to the uterus or fetus, such as deep penetration or rough sex.

If you or your partner have concerns about sexual activity during pregnancy, seek the advice of a healthcare provider or a counselor who specializes in sexual health and relationships.

In conclusion, pregnancy can bring many changes to sexual health and relationships. By communicating openly and honestly with each other and taking steps to maintain sexual health and safety, expectant parents can navigate these changes and maintain a strong and intimate connection during this exciting and transformative time.

# 18.PREGNANCY AND RELATIONSHIPS

Pregnancy is an exciting time for expectant parents, but it can also bring changes and challenges to their relationships. In this chapter, we will explore the ways that pregnancy can impact romantic relationships, friendships, and family dynamics, and offer tips for navigating these changes.

**Impact on Romantic Relationships:**

Pregnancy can bring significant changes to romantic relationships, including changes in sexual desire, physical discomfort or pain during sex, and increased stress and anxiety. Here are some tips for maintaining a strong and healthy relationship during pregnancy:

- Communicate openly and honestly with your partner about your feelings and needs. This can help you both understand and support each other through the changes and challenges of pregnancy.

- Seek out resources, such as books, classes, or counseling, that can help you learn about and prepare for the physical and emotional changes of pregnancy.

- Make time for intimacy and connection outside of sexual activity, such as cuddling, massage, or spending quality time together.

- Take care of your own physical and emotional needs, such as getting enough rest, eating well, and seeking support from friends or professionals when needed.

**Impact on Friendships:**

Pregnancy can also bring changes to friendships, as expectant parents may feel disconnected from friends who are not experiencing similar changes in their lives. Here are some tips for maintaining friendships during pregnancy:

- Communicate openly with friends about your experiences and feelings, and try to include them in your journey as much as possible.

- Seek out friendships with other expectant parents, as they may be better able to understand and support your experiences.

- Be patient with friends who may not be as understanding or supportive, and recognize that their priorities and experiences may be different from yours at this time.

**Impact on Family Dynamics:**

Pregnancy can also bring changes to family dynamics, as expectant parents may need to navigate relationships with parents, in-laws, and extended family members. Here are some tips for managing family relationships during pregnancy:

- Communicate openly and honestly with family members about your experiences and needs, and set clear boundaries if necessary.

- Seek out support from family members who are understanding and supportive, and try to involve them in your journey as much as possible.

- Be patient with family members who may not be as supportive, and recognize that their reactions may be influenced by their own fears or anxieties.

In conclusion, pregnancy can bring significant changes and challenges to relationships. By communicating openly and honestly, seeking out support, and taking care of your own physical and emotional needs, expectant parents can navigate these changes and maintain strong and healthy relationships with their partners, friends, and family members.

# 19. PREGNANCY AND TRAVEL

Traveling during pregnancy can be a great way to relax, connect with loved ones, or experience new cultures before the arrival of your baby. However, pregnancy can also bring certain risks and considerations when it comes to travel. In this chapter, we will explore the potential risks of traveling during pregnancy and offer tips for safe and enjoyable travel.

**Risks of traveling during pregnancy:**

There are several risks associated with traveling during pregnancy that expectant mothers should be aware of, including:

- Blood clots: Pregnant women have an increased risk of developing blood clots, particularly on long flights or car rides.

- Preterm labor: Traveling long distances, particularly by air, can increase the risk of preterm labor.

- Infections: Pregnant women may be more susceptible to certain infections, particularly those transmitted through food or water.

- Limited access to medical care: Traveling to remote or unfamiliar areas may make it difficult to access medical care in the event of an emergency.

**Tips for safe and enjoyable travel:**

Despite these risks, many women are able to travel safely and comfortably during pregnancy. Here are some tips for safe and enjoyable travel:

- Consult with your healthcare provider before making travel plans, particularly if you have any underlying medical conditions or complications.
- Choose your destination carefully, avoiding areas with a high risk of infectious diseases or limited medical care.
- Consider the mode of transportation, particularly if you are traveling by air or car. Look for opportunities to stretch your legs and move around.
- Pack comfortable clothing and shoes that accommodate your changing body.
- Bring plenty of snacks and water to stay hydrated and nourished.
- Plan for rest and relaxation during your travels, taking breaks as needed to rest and recharge.

In conclusion, traveling during pregnancy can be a safe and enjoyable experience with the proper precautions and planning. Be sure to consult with your healthcare provider and take necessary steps to ensure a comfortable and safe journey for you and your baby.

# 20. PREGNANCY AND CULTURAL CONSIDERATIONS

Pregnancy is a universal experience, but cultural practices and beliefs can vary widely across different communities and societies. It's important for expectant mothers to be aware of cultural considerations and how they may impact their pregnancy and childbirth experience. In this chapter, we will explore some of the cultural considerations that pregnant women may encounter.

**Cultural beliefs and practices surrounding pregnancy and childbirth:**

Different cultures have different beliefs and practices surrounding pregnancy and childbirth. For example, some cultures believe that a pregnant woman should avoid certain foods, behaviors, or activities, while others encourage certain practices, such as belly binding or herbal remedies. It's important for expectant mothers to be aware of these beliefs and practices and to discuss them with their healthcare provider to ensure they are safe and appropriate.

Cognitive-behavioral therapy (CBT) is a common type of therapy used to treat PPD and PPA, which focuses on identifying and changing negative thought patterns. Antidepressant medication may also be prescribed in some cases. Support groups, such as postpartum support groups, can provide women with a safe and supportive environment to discuss their experiences and share coping strategies.

**Self-Care Strategies for Preventing and Coping with Postpartum Depression and Anxiety:**

Self-care strategies can be an important part of preventing and coping with PPD and PPA. These can include exercise, relaxation techniques such as meditation or deep breathing, and seeking help from family and friends. Getting enough sleep and maintaining a healthy diet can also be beneficial.

**The Importance of Early Intervention and Seeking Help for Postpartum Depression and Anxiety:**

It is important for women to seek help if they suspect they may be experiencing PPD or PPA. Early intervention can help prevent symptoms from becoming worse, and can promote a faster recovery.

**Recognizing the Signs and Symptoms of Postpartum Depression and Anxiety:**

It is important for new mothers and their loved ones to be able to recognize the signs and symptoms of PPD and PPA. These may include feelings of sadness, anxiety, or irritability, changes in appetite or sleep patterns, and difficulty bonding with the baby. Women with PPA may also experience physical symptoms such as sweating, heart palpitations, or gastrointestinal distress.

**Risk Factors for Developing Postpartum Depression and Anxiety:**

There are several risk factors that may increase a woman's likelihood of developing PPD or PPA. These include a history of depression or anxiety, a lack of social support, stressful life events such as a difficult birth or financial difficulties, and hormonal changes associated with childbirth.

**Treatment Options for Postpartum Depression and Anxiety:**

There are several treatment options available for women who experience PPD or PPA. These include therapy, medication, and support groups.

**Communication with healthcare providers:**

Communication is key when it comes to navigating cultural considerations during pregnancy. Healthcare providers may not be aware of cultural practices or beliefs that are important to their patients, so it's important for patients to bring these up during appointments. This can help providers offer more personalized and culturally sensitive care.

**Cultural Support Systems:**

Many cultures place a strong emphasis on community and support systems during pregnancy and childbirth. This can include family members, friends, or spiritual leaders who offer guidance and support throughout the process. Pregnant women should consider how their cultural support systems can play a role in their pregnancy and childbirth experience.

**Cultural Barriers to Healthcare Access:**

Cultural considerations can also impact access to healthcare during pregnancy. Language barriers, cultural differences in healthcare practices, and lack of understanding or trust in Western medicine can all be barriers to receiving appropriate care.

It's important for healthcare providers to be aware of these barriers and to work with patients to ensure they receive the care they need.

In conclusion, cultural considerations are an important aspect of pregnancy and childbirth. Pregnant women should be aware of cultural beliefs and practices, communicate with their healthcare provider, consider their cultural support systems, and be aware of potential barriers to healthcare access.

By understanding and navigating cultural considerations, pregnant women can have a safe and positive pregnancy and childbirth experience.

# 21. PLANNING FOR FUTURE PREGNANCIES AND BIRTHS

While the current pregnancy is a priority, it's also important to plan for future pregnancies and births. In this chapter, we will discuss some considerations and steps to take when planning for future pregnancies and births.

**Medical History and Evaluation:**

Before planning for future pregnancies, it's important to review your medical history and evaluate any potential risks or concerns. This can include discussing any past pregnancy complications or medical conditions with your healthcare provider. Based on your medical history, your provider may recommend certain screenings or tests before attempting to conceive again.

**Family Planning and Contraception:**

It's important to have a family planning and contraception strategy in place before attempting to conceive again. This can include discussing birth control options with your healthcare provider and deciding on a method that is safe and effective for you.

It's important to remember that some birth control methods may require a waiting period before trying to conceive again.

**Preconception Care:**

Preconception care involves taking steps to optimize your health before attempting to conceive. This can include maintaining a healthy diet and exercise routine, managing chronic medical conditions, and addressing any mental health concerns. Your healthcare provider can offer guidance on preconception care and recommend any necessary interventions.

**Birth Preferences:**

It's important to reflect on your past birth experiences and consider what preferences you may have for future births. This can include discussing pain management options, delivery location, and birth plan preferences with your healthcare provider. It's important to remember that birth preferences may need to be adjusted based on medical concerns or complications.

**Support Systems:**

Having a support system in place during pregnancy and childbirth is important for physical and emotional well-being. Consider who you would like to have as a support person during future pregnancies and births. This can include family members, friends, or a doula.

In conclusion, planning for future pregnancies and births involves a variety of considerations and steps. It's important to review your medical history, have a family planning and contraception strategy, engage in preconception care, consider birth  preferences, and have a support system in place. By taking these steps, you can optimize your health and well-being for future pregnancies and births.

# 22.SUMMARY

This book is a comprehensive guide for women on pregnancy, covering topics such as preparing for pregnancy, the first, second and third trimesters, nutrition and exercise during pregnancy, managing pregnancy complications, emotional and mental health during pregnancy, labor and delivery, postpartum recovery, newborn care, returning to work and parenting, special considerations for pregnancy, baby's development during pregnancy, pregnancy and sexuality, pregnancy and relationships,, pregnancy and travel, pregnancy and cultural considerations, and planning for future pregnancies and births. It provides detailed information on each topic, as well as recommendations and advice from healthcare providers. I hope that this book has been informative and helpful for all readers.

Thank **you** for reading, I really hope this book helped you with your pregnancy  journey. I encourage you to check out my other books, but only if you want to.